Run, in 10 steps

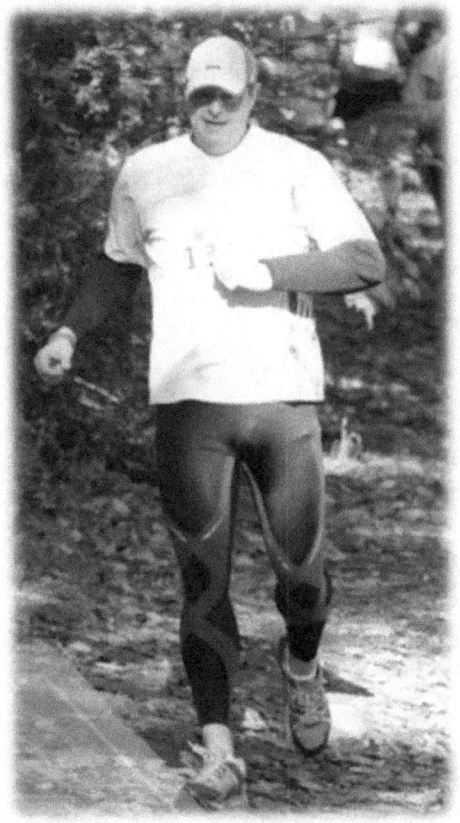

Author Angus Gilbert

Copyright 2014 Angus Gilbert

First Thing

Speak with your Primary Doctor before embarking on any exercise, running program, or applying any of my suggestions.

Take their advice seriously, but work with them so that there is a path to running, even if they say start with a walk, any start is a start.

I am not medically trained. I am not a coach. I run.
Check with your doctor.

About the Author

I am male, 48 years old, and I have been running for 2 1/2 years. I am overweight, have knee pain, diabetes type II, crohn's disease and high blood pressure.

If a runner is someone who can run at least 5k without walking a bit sometimes, then I am not a good runner.

If a runner is someone who can jump out of bed and run every morning, then I am not a good runner.

If a runner is someone who always eats right, I am not a good runner.

If a runner is someone who is always getting faster, I am not a good runner.

If a runner is ... you get the idea.

I run, I don't always enjoy it, and I run 'races' regularly, and sometimes they are really tough, but I always feel good afterwards. My practice or training will have been worthwhile, and I have shown to myself I am fit and strong in body and in mind.

I started running for two reasons;

- My wife started running and booked herself a race as motivation. When I saw her hesitation at times I reluctantly asked 'would you like me to run with you?'
- As a statement to myself that I will not be defined or restricted by my diabetes or crohn's!

I keep running because it challenges me, because it keeps me fit (if not slim), and I can take reward in my achievement post a 'race'.

I have run at least one race every month now for 30 months. I started with 5ks, and have now also run 2 half marathons, a sprint-triathlon (250 yard swim, 10 mile bike ride, then a 5k run), a triple-threat (that is a 1 mile race, followed by a 5k, followed by a half-marathon,) and I ran the Boston Marathon in 2014.

Finishing the Boston Marathon, the year after the bombing will be one of the highlights of my life forever. Talk about a high, and a sense of achievement, nothing tops it.

I should clarify some things for you;

- In that triple threat, I walked most of the half-marathon. I speed walked 13.1 miles and I was not last, close to it, but not last.
- In the Boston Marathon, I crossed the line just before the course was closed down.
- I have finished a 5k with just two people behind me.
- I have been last in my age group on three occasions.

- When training for the Boston Marathon I walked off the long training runs in snow and ice a couple of times, with disgust and fear for what I had taken on.
- I always finish.
- Running is a mind game, more than it is a physical ability.
- My body is fitter, and my mind is stronger.

I have to acknowledge my wife. She got me started with running, and she books most of the next races. She drags me out to run some mornings, and some I drag her out.

We start races together with a fist bump and a kiss, and then she usually finishes a little ahead of me. The Boston Marathon we stayed together, paced, pushed and pulled each through it, and crossed the line holding hands, with exactly the same time down to hundredths of a second.

I also owe a lot to our Boston Marathon Coach Rick Muhr, a simply inspirational human being, thank you Coach.

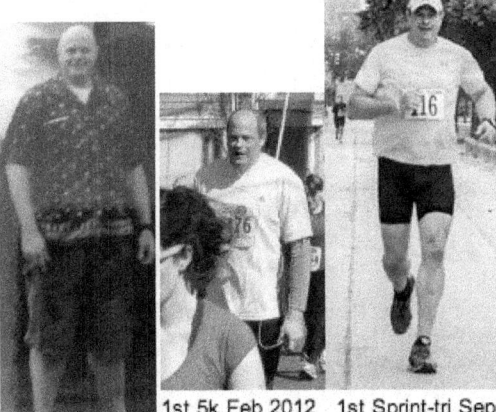

1st 5k Feb 2012   1st Sprint-tri Sep 2013

Pre-Running

Contents

Introduction

Run for you.
Run for your health.
Run to get outside and for your heart.
Run to raise your fitness level.
Run to strengthen you mind and your will power.
Running has never been so popular.

I have the best looking toned legs, sitting right under my large belly. If you want to lose weight with running, then you need to eat properly too, and ideally incorporate some cross-training. I have lost about 20lbs, and can drop 1 to 2lb any week by counting my calories and running.

So why read my book about running when there are so many out there? So many magazines and online sites too?

I am for real, and you can relate to me. The odds are my background and experience will relate more to you and what you do with running, than many other runners who write books or contribute to magazines.

I am betting we are similar, in our physique, fitness levels and challenges. I do not know you, and therefore I cannot personalize this book to your current physical condition or running experience. You need to draw from this book that someone else has been there, this fatty makes it work for him, and has simple, practical and relevant advice to get you started.

This almost 50-year-old guy does it without concern for being last, without regard for the huge amounts of sweat (puddles) he can make. This guy who has been largely inactive for 45 years got up off the couch.

I did it, so you ask yourself again, 'why not me?' I have tried to keep this book short, and such that you can jump to the Checklist if you want. Then look back to the steps and more information when you need.

I have structured this book as follows, starting with **Couch to 5k,** I talk about this training plan or method briefly. This is the best way to start. I then add to that practical experience regarding all the other questions you have, and need answered to get you to your first 5k 'race'.

In the chapter '**My method to get running**', I have addressed things that are going through your head like, where can I run, and I guarantee some you have not come up against yet. Most importantly I start to talk about getting motivated, and staying motivated.

You can jump right to '**The 10 steps**' if you want where I give structure to my method, and present the information you need to start running in easy and concise steps.

In '**More information**' I give you, more information on the topics covered, and a few new ones I thought of, like socks and what to-do and what to expect on race day.

The '**Checklist**' is just that, when you are ready to start, even if it is now, before reading any part of the book, you can go to this checklist. Follow this in sequence, employing the spaces to record the information, and just go running. Being an eBook remember you can print just the checklist pages, to write on.

If you choose to print this book, if you choose '2 pages per sheet' you use half the paper and still be able to read it.

I want to share my experience and to encourage you.

You can do it.

Couch to 5k

The couch to 5k program is the way everyone seems to be getting into running at the moment. There are books, articles, online pieces, entire websites and smartphone applications dedicated solely to guiding you with the couch to 5k program.

It is a simple method; you start with walking and running, with a lot of time walking at first, and slowly reduce the walking while increasing the running.

So you might run for 1 minute, and walk for 4. Next week you would run for 2 minutes, walk 4. Then run for 2 minutes, walk 3. Run 3, walk 3. Get it, you slowly build up to running without stopping?

You do not need buy a 'couch to 5k' book, just Google 'Couch to 5k' and pick a program, or training schedule you like.

The principle does work, it is a very sound method for breaking up running when you are not use to that level of duration or movement. When my wife and I trained for the Boston Marathon, we had a coach assigned through the Charity Group we were running for, and his advice was run for 8 minutes, and walk 1 with any long run. It breaks it up for the legs, and your mind.

I had one problem with the Couch to 5k method, in that I could never quite get rid of the walking part. I would run for 5 minutes and walk 1, next run for 6 minutes and walk 1. Then one day my wife said 'just run will you', and I did.

Form

I have caused myself more frustration and harm by getting hung up on my running form. Run, just put one foot in front of the other and run. It is natural.

Remember you are going for distance, not speed, so do not sprint. Putting one foot in front of the other, that is all you need to visualize.

I have attended a running form class, read numerous articles on the subject, and sort out coaching advice. I did this because I wanted to run faster. This is not why we are running though. To work on form like that takes serious time, training and feedback mechanisms, such as a coach and video recording.

The two periods I really focused hard on my form, and on developing to get more speed, I ended up giving myself a muscle injury. On the last occasion I need some physical therapy to aid recovery.

Just focus on one foot in front of the other, land on your sole and get something of a heel strike, barely a touch. You are running.

The only other thing I will say on form is to keep your head up, and looking forward for many reasons;

- It helps pull your posture straight, and reduces the chance of neck or back ache.
- It allows you to keep on an eye on traffic and surface conditions.
- It keeps the airway more open for improved breathing.

Mind game

This is a mind game, as much as it is a physical challenge. The couch to 5k approach supports that too, the further you can go with running and walking will build your confidence.

You will discover through pushing yourself mentally that when your body appears to be saying 'enough', there is plenty more in your legs, it is your mind saying 'stop'.

I will discuss techniques for handling the mind game.

Go into it knowing it is a mind game and you have a head start, because you will understand you are building confidence. I have finished many a 5k by saying to myself, 'you have done this so many times before'.

Warm-up - stretch

If you read the running magazines or look online, you will find endless and confusing advice and opinion on the topic of stretching before and after a run.

It is very simple, you need to warm up your muscles before shocking them with use. You do this by moving your legs; swing them around, jump and down. You can even walk fast back and forth. Anything that prevents them from going from cold to movement will prevent damage.

Then you stretch after a run to prevent the muscles going cold fast, and snapping back. These are the post stretches I do;

- **Walk.**
  A 10 minute walk is a great stretch and cool down.
- **Calf stretch.**
  Stand with the front half of your feet on a curb stone, and drop your heels, you should feel the stretch in your calves. Hold while comfortable, up to 10 seconds, do 3 times.
- **Hamstring stretch.**
  Put a foot behind you and up, then grab the foot with a hand, and pull it back up as far as is comfortable, you want to just start to feel the stretch in your upper leg. Hold for up to 10 seconds, repeat with the other leg, repeat 3 times.
- **Back stretch.**
  Put one arm straight across your chest, put the other hand on your elbow and pull it in close to your chest. You should feel it in the shoulder. Hold for 10 seconds, do the other arm. Repeat 3 times.
- **Gluteus stretch.**
  Simple toe-touching, you do not need to touch them or be totally straight legged, just feel the stretch in hamstrings and gluteus. Hold for 10 seconds, repeat 3 times.

My method to get running

This is my method, which you could also call my story.

This represents the experience and the detail that goes behind the 10 steps found later on, and you can jump to the 10 steps now and refer back to here if you prefer.

Motivator

You have to find a motivator. I am most fortunate that my motivator is my wife. My boss too has been a motivator at times, he runs Ironman's and at times during a race I visualize telling him on Monday of my time, or my new distance.

You just need someone who you can look forward to receiving a positive response from when you tell them how far you ran/walked, and of your first race.

Your partner, your mother, a colleague, your best friend, your Doctor. Let them know what you are embarking on, and what you need from them, which is just to be positive and encouraging.

Facebook friends can be a motivator at the start. I found that at first when I posted 'Ran 2 miles today, only walked .5 mile' I got likes and positive comments. I found that eventually though it stops, after about 6 or 9 months. I do not post my training runs anymore, but I post every 'RACE DAY' with the location and the distance and that gets some likes.

My wife is my motivator, but not my motivation.

Motivation

Motivation is what gets me from bed into running gear and out the door.

Motivation is what keeps me moving when running. Motivation is why I always finish a race.

You need to find your motivations, my principal ones are:

- **The next run.**
  The closer a run comes, the easier I find it is to do my training runs.
- **My weight.**
  When I have gained back a pound or two, or know I ate too much yesterday, I find it easier to go .
- **The emotion, or high.**
  The feeling after a run definitely motivates me on race day, it is so exhilarating, and to say to myself 'I did it' is great. This has worked too with training runs. When I have got into a rut and not run for a week, I recall the way I feel afterwards, energized, strong and taking care of myself.

- **Location.**

  Location can be a motivator too. A change of scene from my normal training route is always refreshing, but on race day especially. I am lucky, I have to travel for work sometimes, and my wife and I like to travel. One of my favorite runs is an early morning run through the streets of Santiago in Chile.

- **The weather.**

  If you are a sun lover, then get some sun and run. I love the rain, in fact some of my fastest run times have been in the rain! I enjoy a reason to get wet, and splash through muddy puddles.

These are my most common motivations per run stage.

- At the start, actually showing up for the race, or getting out for a training run;

  - Knowing I have done this distance so many times before.
  - Being with my motivator.
  - Knowing I paid money to 'race', and I do not waste money.
  - Because I can, because this is what I do.

- To keep me going during the run.

  - Sight of my wife just ahead.
  - Knowing I have done this before.
  - The count off,
    - On short runs, the phone application MapMyRun tells me the distance covered and therefore to go.
    - On long runs, the application calls out every minute, so I can run for 8 minutes, and walk 1.
  - The thought of yesterday's dessert
  - I think of Jeff Bauman and who lost both legs watching the Boston Marathon,
  - And brave soldiers who never get to run again.

- Finish;

  - Knowing this is only way back to the car or home . I use that one a lot.
  - Listening to music with a good tempo.
  - Cowbells. If you are ever a spectator at a race finish, please ring the runners in with a cowbell, we love it. Especially when the finish is round a corner, you can hear the cowbells ringing you in before you see the finish.
  - Sight of the finish.
  - To get that sense of achievement.

Couch to 5k

It is a simple method; you start with walking and running, with a lot of time walking at first, and slowly reduce the walking while increasing the running.

So you might run for 1 minute, and walk for 4. Next week you would run for 2 minutes, walk 4. Then run for 2 minutes, walk 3. Run 3, walk 3. Get it; you slowly build up to running without stopping.

You do not need buy a 'couch to 5k' book, just Google 'Couch to 5k' and pick a program, or training schedule you like.

Apply this program, and after ever run think about what you have achieved, and how you once thought it beyond your ability.

See the previous section on Couch to 5k for more information.

Sneakers

For your sneakers, you have to go to running store, not a big chain sports shop, but a store that specializes in running. They should insist you step outside and run in the sneakers while they watch you.

I suggest getting some advice before going into a store, so you know if they have a clue. This link is a great guide from Runners World.
http://www.runnersworld.com/shoe-finder/shoe-advisor

My wife has worn those Vibram's finger shoes from day one and they work for her. I am now on my third style of sneaker, after starting with the vibram's.

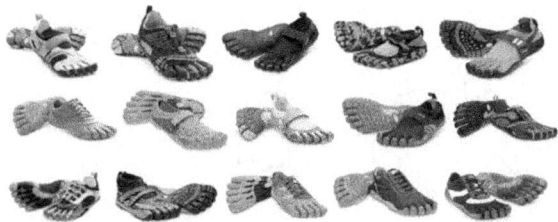

When it comes to running sneakers;

- It may take a few attempts to get to the right pair.
- Get advice.
- Listen to your and feet over time, and not from one run.
- If you need orthotics, get orthotics.
- Change your sneakers every 250 miles.
- Please buy your sneakers from a local specialized store. Once I find a style, I used to buy replacements on line to save money, but you need to support that local store.

Where

You need to find a place to run. A place readily accessible and close to home if you are going to run before work.

Road

For me that place is the road that runs past my house and on towards a lake. I have come to know it very well;

- to the lake and back is 5k,
- to the end of the road and back is 6 miles,
- take a right at the end and loop around is 8 miles.

My road has light to medium traffic, and has a good surface, but no sidewalk! So here are some pointers for running on the road;

- Run towards the traffic.
- Look to make eye-contact with the driver, that way you know they see you.
- Wear bright colors, and as the light fades a reflective top or band, even lights.
- If a cyclist is coming towards you step off the road, stop if you have too. Do not make them move out into traffic to go around you.
- If a car is turning right onto the road you are running on, go behind them or stop. Many a driver does not think to check to the right.

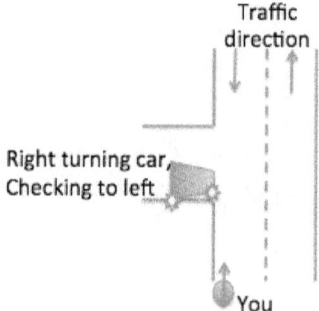

- Watch the cars behind the front car. You may have eye contact with the driver of the first car, while the one behind has not even seen you.
- Be thankful to cars that stop for you.

- Do carry your phone.
- Do carry or wear Id.

I do like to mix it up though for some variety and if I am running in the evening or at the weekend I will either go to local park where there is a one mile loop marked out, or to a State Forest nearby and run the trail.

I have been known to use the track at the local high school on a Sunday morning too.

Grass

Grass is a great surface to run on, probably the best. It is soft and easier on you and your legs. Look out though for hazards, like little piles left by dogs and bad owners.

Rail-Trails

Rail-Trails are one of the best places to run. They usually have a firm but not hard surface, and a wide path. They can be very popular, making running difficult at the busiest times.

Sand

Avoid sand because it's instability creates strain and pull on the joints.

Weather

If it is hot and sunny, be sure to hydrate and if you sweat a lot get some electrolytes, the easiest way to do this is with a sports drink. Note though that you cannot hydrate for a run moments before you start, that is too late. You need to drink plenty of liquids all day long. As I sweat a lot, on the long runs I actually take a salt tablet when I finish, and for half marathons take a couple during the run.

Rain is a personal choice, it can make the road conditions and visibility more difficult, but I love the rain and so I run in it.

I prefer the cold days, and just replace my shorts with running tights, and wear long sleeves shirt, even gloves and a wool hat if necessary.

When there is snow and ice, I would of once said avoid it and use a treadmill. Then I discovered that the hardest thing about the Boston Marathon (for a New Englander) is that because it is in April, you have to do long training runs in the winter, through snow and over ice. I have become more comfortable with these conditions now, and will run through snow and ice where there is a path or sidewalk, but not on the road.

I keep this simple guide on my fridge, so I do not need to think about what to wear.

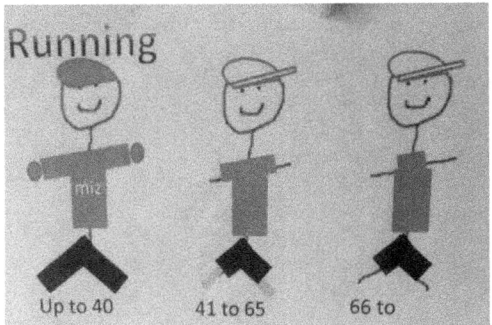

So up to 40 degrees I wear a wool hat, gloves, long sleeved cold weather top, compression tights. 41 to 65 I wear a cap, short sleeve top, shorts and compression socks.

I also have on the fridge two charts I got online; one calculates Wind Chill, and the other Heat Index.

Track

Tracking your runs is a great idea, and there are some advantages. If you track the temperature and what you wore, with how you felt you will get to know what to wear in what conditions. That is how I developed my chart above.

A log allows you to look back and not only see improvements, but just how many miles you have covered since you started, you will be surprised how quickly the miles build up.

At a minimum you must track the distances run in your sneakers. It is of vital importance that you replace your sneakers every 250-300 miles depending on your weight and budget. There is no point in buying the right sneaker, and then continuing to use it when all the support you bought it for has gone.

Mix it up

You are going to get bored, that is if you do not mix it up. What you do while you are running, and what you think about is a personal choice and that will develop over time. I know people who think about their day while running, for me it is a kind of meditation, I think of nothing but the next footstep.

So mix up your runs, and mix up your races.

I once did a 5k that went up a ski-trail (in the fall), through some woods, and then down a fire (access) road. As we started to climb up and through trees I started to think 'what the hell have I taken on'. Then as I came back down through the woods, it was beautiful, the sun was shining and with 500 yards to the end I leapt past my wife, leaping to clear some logs, and with a 'Hello' finished just ahead of her!

We still laugh about the 5k in Edinburgh, Scotland on New Year's day. We did not realize it was organized by a running club. Practically everyone else there was a hard-core runner. I have never, in any other race seen the runners move off so fast at the start, I thought 'shit, where did they all go'. I finished that race with just two people behind me.

To mix up the training runs at home, be prepared to drive when you have the time, because just a little drive can change the scene totally. A park, a field, a quite road, a decent sidewalk, the woods or around a lake.

As for the races, there is a lot of variety, races can come with;

- Beer
- Food
- Live music
- Color paint thrown at you
- Donuts
- Prizes for costumes
- Flat runs
- Trail runs
- Chocolate runs (a favorite)

Next race

Get on line and either Google 5k's in your area, or go to Active.com and book yourself a race. Now you are committed, you have spent some money, and you have another motivation for training. Book it 3 months out from today.

When you have done that run, book another in a months time, and keep booking them.

Simple goals

I actually call the races runs now, as a race implies you have to beat someone and that you have to win or at least place high. I am there to run, not to race anyone. If you goal is to race, then your motivation might suffer after some time.

My three goals of any run have always been;

1) Finish
2) Not be last
3) Not be last in my age group

I have always achieved one and two, and on most occasions number three too. I was given a medal in one race for being first in my age group! Of course I was the only one in my age group.

Race size may affect your goals and motivations. If the run has 100 runners as mine did that day I got the medal, it may be hard to achieve all those goals.

As I pass the half way point in most races I usual develop a new, short-term goal. That is simply that my car is back at the start, and there is only one way to get to it, to run back to it.

Forget pace

You need to be careful of your goals. I started with the simple intent to increase my pace, and I was able to do that as I trained more. Eventually though I plateaued, and I started to get frustrated that my pace was not improving. That is when I started to mess with form and ended up with a minor muscle injury and a lot of frustration.

Perhaps better advice would be change up your training goal from time to time. Right now mine is to build back up the distance and get back into the zone. I can hit a zone after a few miles, where everything is natural and keeping moving is a rhythm, my head is 100% in it. I love the zone.

Pains

You will get some pains, these are to be expected.

Do seek medical advice with any persistent pains, and google them too. Not all Doctors are runners, so you should go prepared with some of your own research ready.

I developed shin splints when I started, then I switched to a shoe with more of a heel and that went away.

As I pushed up my distance while also working on form and speed I developed calf pain, which was resolved with Physical Therapy and switching to a shoe with more arch support.

It may take a while to find the right pair of shoes, but any discarded shoes can become a pair of walking shoes, gym shoes or just a casual pair of shoes.

I suffer with chronic knee pain in my left knee, and the right from time-to-time. It is due to a history of a desk job, crossing my legs and weak muscles around the joint and kneecap. My knee pain was always my biggest excuse for not being able to run.

It did hurt at first, and it can still hurt for about the first half mile, but after that I can run for hours pain free. That is because it is stronger, has a little less weight on it, and you produce more joint fluid and natural pain suppressants as you exercise.

Warm-up – stretch

It is very simple; you need to warm up your muscles before shocking them with use. Move your legs, swing them around, jump and down. You can even walk fast back and forth. Anything that prevents them from going from cold to movement, that can do damage.

Then you stretch after a run, which prevents the muscles going cold fast, and snapping back.

See the other chapter on Warm-up – Stretch for more information, and my exercises.

Techniques to stay moving, and to finish

A lot of people use music to keep them moving, and to distract themselves. Not everyone does though, you need to find out what works for you. Music can be a powerful way to set a pace, or a finishing sprint. My wife listens to music during the whole run, where as I use it in the closing mile, and my boss never listens to music!

When I started I always listened to music, but I tried a week with none, and realized how much beauty of the sound of nature and my own mind I had been missing.

Here are some techniques to keep your moving;

- **Music**
    - Use music as a distraction, to listen to, or to set a pace.
    - Listen to music for a strong finish. As soon as I see the finish I put on 'I love it' by Icona Pop. A stupid song with great energy.
    - I have a Running playlist for when I am on a treadmill, made up of a mix of fast paced music.
- **Markers**
    - You pick an object up ahead, maybe a mailbox and run to that. For the next few minutes that is all you are focused on. Then the next marker.
- **Pacer**
    - A similar paced runner. If you find after a few minutes that you are looking at the back of the same person, then stick with them. Just be careful they do not up the pace or slow right down.
- **Time Counter**
    - On long runs my phone counts off every minute, this allows me to run for 8 minutes, and walk for 1. Thinking to myself 'I can keep this up for two more minutes' works for me.

- **Distance Counter**
  - On short runs my phone tells me how far I have run. I calculate how far is left in my head, this is a great distraction and motivator for me.
- **Images**
  - Then there are the mental images, thinking about those that cannot run, or in a run we once did for fallen soldiers, thinking about what they sacrificed made the run real easy.

In the marathon our coach was at mile 15 and he said to us 'just two more miles and then it is single digits'. We went 'wow, that is great, oh we have this'. Then my mind did the math, 15+2, from 26.2... and by the time I realized that meant there was 11.2 miles to go, we had covered another mile without even realizing it.

The 10 steps

1 Doctor

I am telling you again to check with Doctor first. It is a good idea to know your Couch-to-5k training schedule first, so your Doctor can work with you to suggest modifications if necessary.

2 Motivation

You need motivation to run.
You need to understand why you are getting out there and moving, and why you train.

You need to understand what will keep you moving on your runs.

For my wife her motivation is to beat her age, to challenge the concept of aging. She started with the goal of running a 5k before her 46th birthday. She did that, and has not stopped running since.

My primary motivation is to be ready for the next race. On race day though I have these three goals to keep me moving of;

- Finish
- Not be last
- Not be last in my age group.

I also need to challenge my idea of who I am. For 45 years I saw myself as a couch potato, who could not run. I would say 'I cannot run, I have tried, I physically cannot do it'. Running challenges that, it also ensures the diabetes and crohn's do not define, limit me, or my choices.

3 Book a 5k

Find a 5k that occurs three months after your scheduled Doctor's appointment. Do this by Googling 5ks in your town or state and register. A list of websites that have race information is included in the Useful Links section.

Most runs give you an indication of the terrain and the field size, I suggest you choose flat and with no more than 500 runners.

4 Sneakers

You have to go to running store, not a big chain sports shop, but a store that specializes in running. They should insist you step outside and run in the sneakers while they watch you.

I suggest getting some advice before going into a store, so you know if they have a clue. This link is a great guide from Runners World.
http://www.runnersworld.com/shoe-finder/shoe-advisor

5 Find someone/ group

You can do this on your own, but it will be much easier with someone else. That someone could also be a group that runs once a week from the running store for example.

My wife and I never stay together during a run or race because our paces are different. We always start together, and whoever finishes first cheers the other to the finish.

She is a reason I cannot dodge the race.

She kicks me out of bed some mornings to go run together, and I am sure to return the favor some mornings. We made an agreement; if the other says 'lets go run', you are not allowed to refuse.

6 Couch-to-5k

See the earlier section on Couch to 5k.

7 Experiment

have You have to find what works for you when running threw experimentation. Race day is not the time to experiment, you leave your routine alone on race day. Use your training days to find out what works.

When running I suggest experimenting with these things (at least);

- **Music**
  Experiment running with music, no music, and different styles of music.
- **Phone carrying**
  If you are going to run with your phone, try with it in your hand, and if that does not work try it in a runner's waist bag.

- **Ending music**
  Does a specific tune for the last few minutes help you finish strong, even sprint in? Think energy, tempo and motivating power or lyrics.
- **Headphones cable**
  Try your headphones down your front, behind your neck, and even inside the front of your shirt.
- **MapMyRun**
  Experiment with different feedback (voice) options with MapMyRun, maybe 'pace' will motivate you like 'distance' motivates me.
- **Sunglasses**
  Is running with sunglasses comfortable for you? If not could different sunglasses work better?
- **Marker running**
  Does running to the next marked help you keep moving during the run?
- **Rubbing**
  Ask yourself after your runs, is anywhere chaffing? If so is the answer to try a different (top, shorts, shoe) or is it to apply some lubrication where it runs (chamois butter, glide, petroleum jelly).
- **Tops, Shorts**
  Are you clothes comfortable? Not restricting any area, or causing any friction.
- **Motivations**
  Which motivations are working for you during the run? File them away in your mind for future use.

- **Mind**

  Was your mind in the run?

  Did your thoughts encourage or question you?

  How can you keep your mind focused; for me that is to focus on the next step, and the next step, or a marker.

8 Race day

Runs, not races

I have started calling them runs in my head, and not races. Races imply winning, and that can be intimidating for many of us. It is a run for 99% of the participants.

I feel better dwelling on finishing ahead of 50 runners, than on finishing 500 places behind a racer!

See the section Race Day under More Information for Race Day guidance on;

- Breakfast and carbs
- Hydration and Toilets
- Post race
- Bib Placement
- Photographers
- Headphones, Strollers and Dogs
- Running community and Etiquette
- Distance and Time

9 Positive

Mix it up

There are so many races to choose from now, you can easily mix it up for variety and challenge. Keep yourself stimulated.

Last Fall I wore one red sneaker and one yellow for every run, to match with fall colors, (they had the same miles on them). It made a lot of other runners want to talk to me, I loved it, and it made every run different for a while.

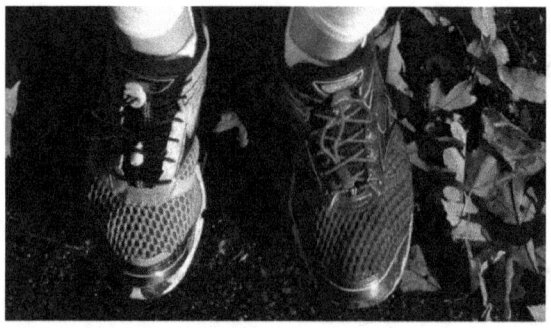

I did a sprint-triathlon last year for a change, that is 250 yards in a pool, 10 mile bike ride, and then a 5k. That motivated my training to a whole new level.

Never be embarrassed, never make excuses

I used to be embarrassed to talk about my runs at work, I thought I was not running fast enough. After I had to walk much of a half-marathon I felt I was a fraud, and I did not want to talk about it.

Remember, every time you get out and run, you are passing everyone on the couch.

You are running for your goals, no one else's.

I have three colleagues, younger than me, that tell me they started running with Couch-to-5k, all because of me.

Find the positive post a run

After your races, and not necessarily right away, find the positive from that run. Write it down next to your alarm clock and on a note in your sneakers. To recapture that moment is another motivation to get up and run, to train.

Know what keeps you moving

Work with your training runs to find out what keeps you moving. Refer back to the section on this for ideas.

Mind

Running is a mind game, far more than a physical game. Every time you run you are training your mind as much as you are the body.

Your mind will say 'Done', and you will think it is your legs 'talking' Push through and you will usually find there is more in your legs. Your mind is just trying to quit early.

That is why you have to work on every step above.

I get past the first mile knowing, based on my experience that it gets better after that.

I keep going because I have done it before. I push through the days when I hear 'enough' because I know from experience I can beat that.

Keep your mind in the run.

There will be bad runs, bad days. Forget them, and run again the next time. They are normal.

10 Book next race now

Always be booking your next race to stay motivated and focused. I always have a run for coming months booked. At least one every month.

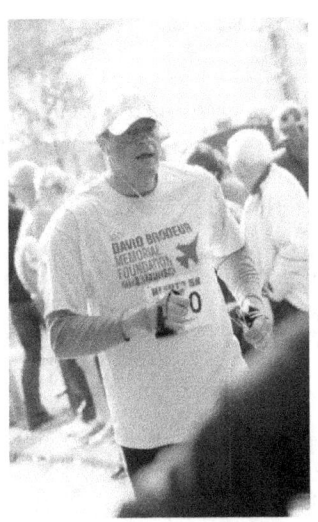

More Information

Running Alone

Whether you are running alone, with someone or in a group you should always have identification on you. You can carry your driver's license in your hand, in a waist bag, or in a phone case. The best form of identification though is a wrist band, check out these at Road ID.
www.RoadId.Com

If you are running alone, somewhere new or remote, tell you motivator where you are running. My wife's trick is to have MapMyRun set so I can see where she is running real-time.

Sneakers

You have to go to a running store for your running sneakers, and not a big chain sports shop, but a store that specializes in running. They should insist you step outside and run in the sneakers while they watch you.

I suggest getting some advice online before going into a store, that way you will know if they have a clue. This link is a great guide from Runners World.
http://www.runnersworld.com/shoe-finder/shoe-advisor

You must change your sneakers every 250-300 miles, because they are losing their support by this stage.

Lacing

For running 5ks, and I have found longer runs too, it does not matter how you lace your sneakers, so long as you are comfortable and there is no rubbing.

If you really want to get into the topic of lacing, this is the only site to visit,
http://www.fieggen.com/shoelace/lacingmethods.htm

Socks

I wear compression socks if I am wearing shorts. I strongly believe based on experience that they help with endurance and recovery. I put (clean) ones back on after long runs to aid with recovery. The only exception is when I wear compression tights in the winter, then I am getting all the compression I need, although I have worn both on some very cold days.

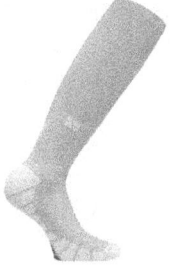

Shorts

Ideally you need shorts that wick sweat, and for us guys give you some support.

On longer runs I wear underwear too, for that increased support. The matter of shorts length is purely a personal choice.

On the longer runs I also apply some chamois butter (as used by cyclists) into my crotch to prevent soreness or chaffing.

Tops

To start wear any short sleeved shirt. When you can though move to a proper running (technical) shirt, they are so comfortable, and wick so well I actually wear them casually in place of cotton shirts now.

Many races include a shirt, and usually now a technical shirt. You will find that before long you have acquired a small collection of shirts you can train and run in.

On longer runs I wear nip guards. If you start running much further than 5k I strongly suggest them for men. It tends not to be a problem for women as they are wearing a tight fitting sports bra, but for us guys the nipples will rub against the tops. After my first half marathon I was bleeding (slightly) from my left nipple.

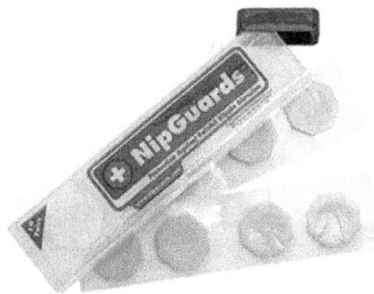

As you run further you will find what rubs, and can then pretreat that area, for example I have to apply some Glide to my wife's back where her sports bra sits.

Hats

Just like the top, you really need a running hat that will wick away sweat. You can tell if it is the real deal by the underside of the brim. It should be dark to reduce reflection onto your face and eyes.

If your winters are cold, you will need a warmer one too.

Sunblock and Sunglasses

My wife rarely runs without sunglasses and some sunblock. I never run with sunglasses, but on sunny days I do apply sunblock to my nose, top of my ears, cheeks and back of my neck.

I have a friend who has run outside his whole life, and they just removed the tops of his ears before the skin cancer spread!

Tights

I love to run in compression tights, I find them very comfortable, but they are expensive. They definitely help me go a little further, and to have a little more stamina, with better recovery.

They are too hot though to wear in the summer for me.

Books and Magazines

I suggest subscribing to a Running magazine for just a year. They tend to repeat the same ideas and advice through a full year. Unless you are really into the very latest trend, technology or runner stats you will learn all the key information in that one year.

Many of the magazines also have a Facebook page, which releases the articles for free, albeit some weeks after the magazine was published.

Books are a personal choice, I have read several on different aspects of running, and one only has really stuck with me. It is about the mind game of any endurance event, it is called The Champion's Mind by Jim Afermow.

Gels

There are so many gels to choose from, and all the big names work. For 5ks though you probably do not need them. I have stopped using gels, even on my long runs. For the long runs now I top up with peanut butter individual serving sachets and/or EFS.

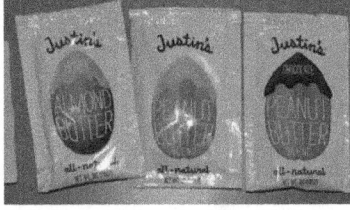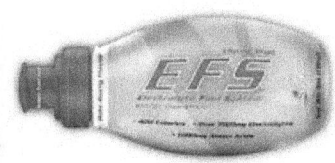

I have used a gel for a kick start before a 5k where I still felt asleep or not into it, but I recently switched though to Organic applesauce, it works just as well and is all natural.

Sports drinks

I am not a fan of most sports drinks because in my opinion, they are a lot of chemicals, but they do work. Again for a 5k you should not need much post run. On longer runs where the water stops have Gatorade, I take a Gatorade, then a water and pour the water into the Gatorade to water it down. Again, it does work, and on the run it is right there being offered to me.

There are other options too; organic ones, vegan ones, and plenty of recipes online to make your own.

Protein

After any exercise you should be getting some extra protein to protect your muscles. It does not have to be some expensive protein shake or drink though. You cannot absorb more than 20g of protein at a session anyway, so why get a 30g bar?

Simply the best protein source post a run is some chocolate milk.

Keys (house or car)

When you go running you are going to need to carry either your car, or house keys. When I have driven somewhere, I shut the house keys up in the glove compartment, and just carry the car key.

For a 5k, I just carry my keys in a hand. On a longer run I wear a belt beg and put them in there with my phone.

I did trade in my old key ring loop for one from EMS that allows me to quickly unclip either my house keys, or car key so I do not have to wind them off those metal rings, and back on afterwards.

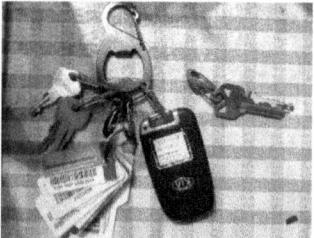

Technology

From what I can see, the racers where GPS watchers, and us runners use an application on our smartphone. For me that is MapMyRun. Not only does it track your run, but it also provides detailed information online if you want to see detailed information your gradient, splits and other data.

The voice feedback options are great for motivation, it has a lot more options than giving you your distance or time at intervals you predetermine, which is all I use.

Every now and again though I like to unplug and run with none of it; no technology, no record of my distance or pace, just run.

How you use technology is your personal choice, for me it provides feedback as I run, which I record for tracking purposes, and of course it gives me my finishing song to come in strong.

Treadmills

Treadmills, I hate them. They do work though for continuing to run when the weather sucks (including too hot). I cannot watch a TV or read when on one, as many people do. I can listen to music, so on goes the tunes with tempo and energy. I think the furthest I have gone a treadmill is 6 miles.

People will tell you that if you put a small gradient on the treadmill it will be just like running outside. That is just not true. You might be better off with a fan in your face to try and simulate running through the air resistance that occurs when you really move forward, rather than run on the spot.

As far as I am concerned treadmills are a necessary evil, I do use them, but try to avoid them.

Car Seats

You are going to be getting back into your car sweaty, so bring a large towel, preferably a beach towel to put over the seat.

I purchased some nice covers recently made just for this purpose. They slot on and off the seats easily. I just put it on after a run, and remove it when I get home. I also bring it if I am in someone else's car. I got mine from www.SeatShield.com

Travel

Sticking to your training and/or nutrition plan can be difficult when travelling. Here are some tips I use;

- Bring with you or purchase on arrival healthy snacks to beat mini-bar and vending machine temptations; 100 calorie almond bags are my favorites, and some dried fruit.
- Ask at the hotel front desk where is a good and safe location to run, starting out from the hotel.
- If you intend to use the hotel's treadmill, have a plan B ready. Then if the treadmill is busy, you just ride the bike (for example) without a hesitation or chance to change your mind.
- If you cannot sleep, or you wake early, go and work out. I once ran 3 miles on a treadmill at a San Jose hotel at 3 in the morning. I had no trouble sleeping after that.

- Listen to your body. On day 1 and when jet lag typically hits you. On those days I set my alarm for the latest time possible to just get ready and leave. If I do wake earlier though, then I exercise.
- If your record your runs on a phone application, add a temporary international data plan to your service before you leave.
- To minimize luggage, a running shirt can be worn socially at night, then for a run the next day.
- Of course I take the gym towels, well the better ones at least.

Stinky sneakers and clothes

If you find your running clothes are retaining an unwanted odor after washing, you can buy 'sports' versions of most detergents which do work. I do not use it every wash, just periodically.

The one drawback of technical clothing is it's potential to retain odors due to the tightly woven fabrics, which are great for wicking and everything else, but not so smell loses.

This is what I use to keep my sneakers smelling fresh.

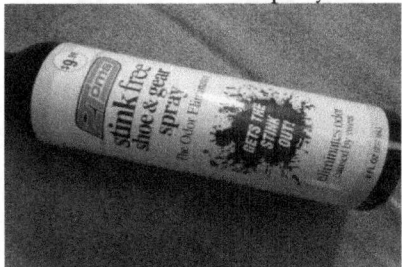

Race day

Breakfast and Carbs

For 5ks your diet is not so important, you do not need to carbo load the night before. You should eat a normal breakfast, which for me is slice of toast with peanut butter. That is a good combination of fast and slow release carbohydrates.

Many runners swear by a morning coffee for a boost, I actually stay away from it on race day as it can clear me out.

Hydration and Toilets

You should be hydrating all the time, as gulping water down just before a race is too late to be of benefit.

There will be some toilets at the event, typically those outside plastic ones. Just as every race has toilets, every race never has enough, so get in line early. If you are hydrating through the day and every day, and not just before the race that should help a little with the need to go.

Post race

After the run be sure to get some electrolytes and protein, with some water, this is easiest done with a sports drink, and a protein drink or bar.

I recommend bringing a bottle of water and leaving it in your car. I have done two races where they actually run out of water for the finishers. That is a terrible way to treat runners, and those are two races I will never repeat.

Bib Placement

Place your bib anywhere on your front. That could be on your shorts or on your top. You will learn after a couple of runs if where you are positioning it catches your arms, or headphones cable.

The photographs that any event photographers take of you will be identified to you by the bib number, and they do not take your picture from behind! So bib on the front, and when you spot a photographer, ensure your arms are not blocking the bib.

Photographers

Look out for the official photographers as you run the race, they often were bright vests, and are the ones with big expensive cameras standing on the road or trail.

Make sure your bib is visible as they need a clear shot of the number to identify you. This might mean briefly mean you need to stop swinging or holding your arms across your front for example.

Headphones, Strollers and Dogs

You will see that some races say 'no headphones', they may also say no baby strollers and no dogs. You will find all three at almost any race. Wear your headphones if you want, I have never been told to remove mine, I think it might be a liability statement on the part of the organizers.

You only tend to see the odd dog with a runner on trial runs, but almost every race has baby strollers. They used to annoy me but you know what, maybe that is their motivation.

In my experience the people with the baby strollers are strong runners, and I think only once I have found myself trying to pass one. If the dog is on a leash then no problem, and that is from someone who is allergic to dogs.

Running community and Etiquette

The running community of your fellow runners are a great bunch. Everyone is there to run, and are happy to help and encourage each other. My wife finished her first half marathon with two strangers she found she was matching pace with about half way through. They started talking, ran together, and now stay in touch.

Just after starting the Boston Marathon I said to my wife, 'I lost a pin already, my bib only has three', and this runner next to me produced a spare pin from her waist bag and gave it to me.

Do try and be considerate;

- If you are passing someone and it is crowded say 'on your left', or right.
- If you are going to be walking, move towards the edge. I slammed into the back of someone once who just stopped in the middle of the road.
- Thank the volunteers and the Police.
- If you have a slow pace, move back in the starting pack.
- Give encouragement to others, whether you are passing them, they are passing you or they are coming back (having already reached the half-way point).
- Have fun, and spread fun.

Distance and Time

If you track your distance and pace with an application or device, I guarantee you will get a different result to the posted times. Courses are measured to the closet edge, so when you turn a corner several people out from the road's edge, you are some feet away from where the course was actually measured right up against that edge. You just a gained a small amount of distance. MapMyRun always says I ran further than the course distance.

I am not sure why timing can be off, but it is usually close. When looking at your results note that;

- **Gun time** is measured from the when the race starts to when you cross the finish. If you are a few seconds back from the start line, you will get a few extra seconds on your time.
- **Chip time** is when you crossed the start to when you crossed the finished, that is the time you are interested in. Most, but not all races use chips.

The results will show your position in your group, that is by sex and age, if you are interested in that.

There is usually a mechanism to challenge a time if you disagree with it. I did this once, and they promptly changed the time. I believe what they do is look at the finish photos to see what runners (and their times) you finished around.

Rest days and Recovery

Your Couch-to-5k program should indicate what days to rest in your training schedule. Do rest, as some recovery time is important to permit recovery and growth. Resist any temptation to run on those days.

Memories

Please keep every race bib. My wife has every one, each with the date and her time written on it. I only started keeping them recently, and wish I had them all.

These are some of my most memorable races, now you too can go make some memories.

The first

We arrived with 3 hours to spare for our first 5k race, so we went into a diner to grab some breakfast, which had been the plan. I then consumed eggs benedict with hash, toast and it came with oatmeal! Do I need to explain why that was a mistake?

We were both over dressed, as I had dressed for the weather when we got there, and not the weather hours later, or for my body temperature when running. I over sweated, and puffed a lot. I look absolutely awful in the photos, although why they placed a photographer at the top of hill just before the end I do not know, we all looked terrible I think.

Cleveland

We did a 5k in Cleveland, which was their inaugural and it turned out to be their last race. We showed up the day before to pick up our bibs as advertised, and no one was there! We went back the next morning though ready to run.

The organizers where there, with bibs and barely a hundred runners; we ran along the waterfront, and it was very beautiful and pleasant. They gave out some prizes afterwards for best times like usual.

Then they had some random drawn prizes, with prizes from their primary sponsor, a chocolate firm. Well, with that small a crowd, my name was called and I bounded up to the front like they wanted to give me the gold medal. My random drawing large candy bar remains a favorite (and rare) race day prize.

Hot Chocolate, Chicago

The Hot Chocolate races are a lot of fun, and we have a done a couple now. They give out chocolate at every opportunity including at the expo, when you are in line for something. It is the only race I have seen that have three tables at the finish marked 'Water', 'Gatorade' and 'Chocolate'.

They are some of best organized races I have attended, and at the end you get a mug of hot chocolate with lots of goodies to dip in it

This was our first big crowd though with 30,000 runners. This was a cold Chicago morning, and we had to get into corals staged by our paces. From the time of the start to our coral getting to the front, was 45 minutes. We were cold, very cold.

Rock and Roll, Las Vegas

We have run Rock and Roll half marathons in Las Vegas and Seattle. These races too are very well organized with storage bags, staged starts, live music every mile, and a large expo before the race.

What can beat though running the Las Vegas strip at night? You start about 6pm as the sun is going down, and they literally shut down the strip, you run past all the casinos, out past the older casinos and sites, past Wedding Chapels where about 30 couples of runners paused to get married, before setting off again.

There are mobs of drunken people on the sidewalks, on the footbridges happy to cheer you on. Then you finish in front of the Bellagio!

This was our second half marathon, and we figured we could walk the mile back to our hotel, having walked from the hotel to the start! If anyone had shot a video of us I am sure it would have gone viral, as I struggled to lift a leg just 4 inches onto the curb.

Triple Threat

There is a run in Rockland, MA every year. They offer a 1 mile race, a 5k, and a half-marathon. You can run any one of the races or register for the triple threat and do all three, back to back.

Last year we did the half marathon, our first. We found it to be a beautiful course, with several parts running right next to beaches and waterfront. It is one the hilliest courses we have done though, and the last mile is all up hill.

We decided to go back this year and do the triple threat. I was not feeling well, and the morning of the race I had diarrhea two hours before the start, and was vomiting an hour before the start. I could not eat any breakfast, because it made me too nauseas.

I refused to be beaten though, and I know that some of best runs have been when I have felt unwell before hand, I have no explanation for that!

I took a couple of Imodium to calm things down, and we set off on the 1-mile. As I ran that I was thinking, oh my god, there is no way I can do the half, this will be the first race I do not finish. I had to run through the finish line and straight to the port-a-potties. I texted my wife and told her to go, don't wait.

I ran from the toilet and straight through the start line of the 5k, at the back of the group. A mile in I started to run/ walk. Then my mind game changed, I started thinking, 'I will not be beaten, I will walk the damn half-marathon if I have to'.

I finished the 5k, grabbed a banana and a water. I told my wife I would be okay, I will finish. I ate half the banana and we set off on the half-marathon.

I walked, well speed walked 13.1 miles and finished ahead of about 5 people.

Mt Wachusset

We did a 5k at Mt Wachusset, which is a Massachusetts state park, and ski mountain in the winter.

We went up ski trails, along trail paths through tress, and then back down through the trails. I loved it, it was so beautiful, I bounced pass with my wife just before the end and yelled 'Hello'.

I wonder if I might be more of a trail runner?

The Boston Marathon 2014

It is hard for me to compare Marathons as I have only run one, that is Boston. When the bombs went off in 2013, I was watching live and within minutes I had declared to my wife 'I will run the marathon next year, no bomber will take running from us, or attack our city'.

The Boston course is most unusual, involving several towns that all have to give permission and work with the organizers. All the other big marathons run within one city.

The route is bizarre too, it actually drops significantly in the first few miles, and if you are not careful your quads do not work later on because of it.

Heartbreak hill is well named, and when I ran it earlier on a 20 mile training run, I was dry-heaving so hard at the end a passerby gave me a bottle of water!

The roads have potholes, train tracks, islands, there can be snow on the ground, or it can be a heat wave.

The crowds are unbelievable and a million of them turn out along the route. Co-workers and friends called out to us in the early miles, I stopped briefly at Wellesley college (an all-girl college) to kiss one of the students. I ran up Heartbreak hill with this kid who came out of the crowd to get in my face and scream 'you got this, you can do it, you are Boston Strong'.

We took frozen ice sticks from a kid who could not of been older than 5 at the top of Heartbreak hill. Strangers handed out towels that they had in buckets of ice.

I turned down the offer of beer from students several times along the route. I high-fived a Boston Cop with Fenway in the background.

Then we turned onto the last 200 yards, hours after the champions had come and gone, not long before the course would start closing down. The crowds were still there, yelling, screaming, the noise was incredible.

If I do not run it next year, I will be there either volunteering or cheering runners home.

Useful links

General Running Resource
Runners World
http://www.runnersworld.com/

Runners World, on Facebook
https://www.facebook.com/RunnersWorld

Shoe Finder
http://www.runnersworld.com/shoe-finder/shoe-advisor

Race Finder
Active.com
http://www.active.com/

Racewire.com
http://racewire.com/events.php

Runners World Race Finder
http://www.runnersworld.com/race-finder

Couch-to-5k
Cool Running
http://www.coolrunning.com/engine/2/2_3/

c25k.com
http://www.c25k.com/

c25k.com, on Facebook
https://www.facebook.com/C25Kplan

Running for Beginners

http://www.runningforbeginners.com/

Post Run Stretches
http://www.fitsugar.com/Post-Run-Stretches-2537378

http://www.sparkpeople.com/resource/fitness_articles.asp?id=1565

MapMyRun
http://www.mapmyrun.com/

Identification
http://www.roadid.com/
www.IdentifyYourself.com

Pace Calculator
http://www.coolrunning.com/engine/4/4_1/96.shtml

Calorie Calculator
http://www.coolrunning.com/engine/4/4_1/94.shtml

Heat Index
http://images.usatoday.com/weather/photos/humid.gif

Chill Index
http://www.atmos.colostate.edu/wx/fcc/images/windchart.png

Car Seat Covers
www.SeatShield.com

Next

CHECKLIST
Use this checklist to get started, please write on the pages.
Check back to earlier sections for more information.

1 Doctor
[Name]   _____

[Number]

_____

Make an appointment and meet with your Doctor before starting.
[Appointment Date / Time]

_____

2 Motivation
List out your goals below.
Which are going to motivate you to train, and which to finish runs?

Motivation

_____

_____

Keep moving

_____

_____

Finish

_____

_____

3 Book a 5k

Find a 5k that occurs three months after your scheduled Doctor's appointment above. Do this by Googling 5ks in your town or state and register. A list of websites that have race information is included in the Useful Links section.

Most runs give you an indication of the terrain and the field size; I suggest you choose flat and with no more than 500 runners.

[Race name] _____
[Race location]

[Race date and time] _____

[Parking] _____

[Bib / Packet pickup] _____

4 Sneakers

Use Google again, or Google maps to find local running shops and go ask for help buying a pair of sneakers.

[Store name] _____
[Store location]

[Store hours] _____

[Date going to store] _____

Obviously while at the store, purchase any other gear you need.

5 Find someone/ group
[Make a list of friends who might run with you]
[and ask them]

Name_____ Answer _____
Name_____ Answer _____
Name_____ Answer _____
Name_____ Answer _____
Name_____ Answer _____
Name_____ Answer _____

Or ask about local running groups at the running store

6 Couch to 5k
Look up Couch to 5k online, and establish you training plan.

Now get out and run, this will be hardest time ever. After this you will always be able to look back and say 'I went out that first time, with no experience, and did it, I can do it again'

Take the positive and motivation from every run, and remember you are passing everyone on the couch.

7 Experiment
[Music while running] Yes_/_ No
[Music to end with] Yes_/_ No
[Phone/ MapMyRun counts off distance] Yes_/_ No
[Phone / MapMyRun count off by time/ splits] Yes_/_ No
[Run to next marker] Yes_/_ No

8 Race day

Do not change anything about your routine on race day, not your running gear, not your form, nothing. This is not the time to experiment.

Warm up before.

Stretch afterwards.

Race day has come, you did it, you ran because you had already done this in training. You had the mind game under control and kept moving for 5k, great job.

[Remind yourself why you did it]

_____

[Who are you telling about it?]

_____

_____

_____

[What is your tip to yourself for next time?]

_____

_____

9 Positive

[What positive did you get from this run?]

_____

_____

10 Book next race now.

Find another race about 30 days after this one, and register for it now. Carry on running.

Further, inspiration

The most inspirational people to me in running, after my wife are the incredible Hoyt's. The love in that father's eyes, and the joy on his son's face move me every time. I look at them and ask, what was my excuse again?

From the Team Hoyt website

Yes You Can!

In the spring of 1977, Rick Hoyt told his father, Dick Hoyt, that he wanted to participate in a 5-mile benefit run for a Lacrosse player who had been paralyzed in an accident. Far from being a long-distance runner, Dick agreed to push Rick in his wheelchair and they finished all 5 miles, coming in next to last. That night, Rick told his father, "Dad, when I'm running, it feels like I'm not handicapped."

This realization was just the beginning of what would become over 1,000 races completed, including marathons, duathlons and triathlons.

http://www.teamhoyt.com/

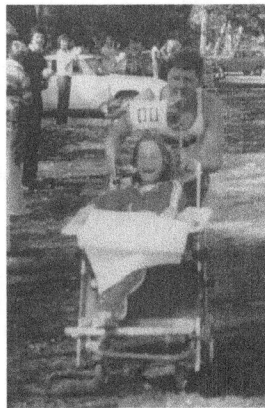 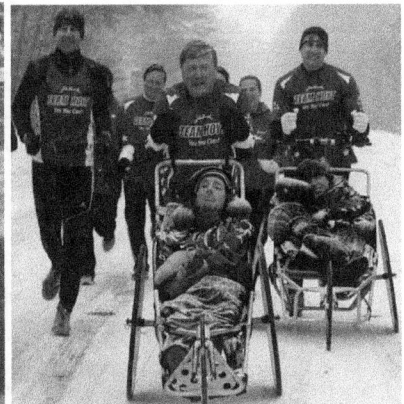

www.ingramcontent.com/pod-product-compliance
Lightning Source LLC
Chambersburg PA
CBHW070608290526
45790CB00002B/835